APPROACHES TO CERVICAL CANCER PREVENTION AND DETECTION

By

Dr. Thomas H. Osborn

Table of contents

cancer. According to a study on ethnic minority women in the UK, there are a number of obstacles to screening, including low perceived risk, lack of understanding, anxiety, humiliation, and shame. Socioeconomic barriers, linguistic limitations, and a weak grasp of health and disease were discovered in one study looking at the obstacles faced by Haitian women. For Black American women in the US, cervical cancer mortality is disproportionately higher. Cervical cancer preventative vaccinations have been available since 2006. In undeveloped nations where resources might not be accessible for routine screening as well as in communities with higher mortality rates, vaccination can reduce the number of cancer deaths.

Dr. Thomas H. Osborn

Part - 1

Chapter 1

Etiology

According to recent studies, the majority of sexually active individuals have contracted the human papillomavirus (HPV) at some time in their lives. There are more than 130 different varieties of HPV that are known, and 20 of those have been linked to cancer. As men are not checked outside of study procedures, the prevalence of HPV-related cervical dysplasia is solely known in women. The most often discovered HPVs in invasive cervical cancer are HPV 16 and 18. Population-based research on HPV prevalence reveals that high-risk HPV is most prevalent in young adults under 25, while cervical cancer mortality peaks between 40 and 50. Cervical illness caused by HPV in women under 25 is typically self-limiting, according to studies. Co-infected individuals may have a lower chance of spontaneous clearance and developing cancer. Age at first sexual contact, multiple sexual partners, smoking, herpes simplex, HIV, co-infection with other genital illnesses, and oral contraceptive usage are risk factors for HPV and cervical cancer. Skin-to-skin contact, such as that experienced during sexual activity, hand-to-genital organ touch, and oral sex, are all methods of transmitting HPV.

Dr. Thomas H. Osborn

Epidemiology

Each year, cervical cancer claims more than 500,000 new lives worldwide. The annual death toll from cervical cancer is about 250,000 women. Every year, over 4000 women in the United States die from cervical cancer. The death rate is significantly higher among Black Americans, Hispanics, and women living in low-resource areas. An infection brought on by a sexually transmitted virus, or HPV, is the cause. Women who have not had a screening in the previous five years or have not received continuous follow-up after discovering a precancerous lesion have a greater death rate from cervical cancer. According to current trends, women most in danger of death may be less likely to get vaccinated against a disease like cervical cancer.

Pathophysiology

The underlying factor in cervical cancer is HPV. High-risk HPV 16 and 18 are to blame for more than 75% of instances. Although there are more than 500,000 instances of HPV diagnosed each year, the majority are low-grade infections that cure on their own within two years. Several carcinogenic variables, such as those mentioned above, accelerate the progression of high-grade lesions and cancer.

Dr. Thomas H. Osborn

Chapter 2

History and physical

Early on, cervical cancer patients are frequently asymptomatic. „, the majority of the, the majority of the acquires, the. The..,. Sexual history includes inquiries regarding post-sexual bleeding and discomfort during sex. The history includes inquiries regarding prior STDs, the total number of partners over a person's lifetime, prior HPV infection, prior HIV infection, prior tobacco usage, and if the patient has previously had an HPV vaccination. Menstrual cycles, unusual bleeding, chronic vaginal discharges, irritations, and cervical lesions should all be brought up when speaking with women. A thorough assessment of the exterior and internal genitalia must be part of the physical examination. Exam results in women with cervical cancer may show a friable cervix, lesions, erosions, bleeding during the inspection, or a fixed adnexa.

Evaluation

Pap testing is advised to start at age 21, according to the United States Preventive Services Task Force (USPTF). Around age 30, Pap smear cytology is combined with HPV testing. For women who continue to receive routine screenings and those at low risk for cervical cancer, screening is advised every three years. Cytology examinations with HPV testing can be done every five

Dr. Thomas H. Osborn

years on women over the age of 30. Women with low-risk status and regular normal screenings are advised to stop cervical cancer cytology and HPV testing at age 65, according to the Level A guideline. There is no need for further screening for women who have undergone a complete abdominal hysterectomy, which included cervix removal, for benign illness.

Individuals who have been given an invasive illness diagnosis need to undergo a thorough staging workup. There are numerous ways to stage a patient according to the International Federation of Gynecology and Obstetrics (FIGO) staging protocol. Traditionally, this was based on the local extent of the tumour, which might be assessed with a pelvic examination, cystoscopy, proctoscopy, chest x-ray, and/or intravenous urography in addition to routine blood tests (CBC, CMP, etc.). More recently, new imaging techniques, including MRI and PET scans, were permitted for staging. A good tool for identifying local tumour extension is a pelvic MRI. It can also be used to measure the response of tumors. PET scans are more sensitive than CT for the identification of nodal and visceral metastases. This is crucial because nodal illness can have a significant impact on the prognosis.

Treatment/Management

Women under the age of 25 are treated conservatively for precancerous lesions. Most aberrant results in women under 25 are caused by low-risk cervical dysplasia and will go away on their own. Colposcopy assesses lesions suspected of being at higher risk or having persistent, abnormal cytology. They are handled in accordance with the results. High-risk lesions are treated according to size, location, and staging, whereas low-risk lesions may be followed and reevaluated more regularly. Small and shallow precancerous lesions are treated with cryotherapy or excision. Conization, laser, or the Loop Electrosurgical Excision Process (LEEP) are utilized to treat lesions that are more severe and include the endocervical canal. The squamocolumnar junction may be better visible with LEEP, and there may be less bleeding in the outpatient environment.

Staging is the next stage in care after an invasive cancer diagnosis to determine the course of treatment. Staging is determined by examination findings, tissue findings, imaging data, and reported signs and symptoms. The size, depth, and presence of symptoms that the cancer has spread to other organs determine the grade. Surgical resection is frequently used to treat early-stage illness and can take the form of anything from a conization to a modified radical hysterectomy. .... in. Conization or trachelectomy may be a choice for women with early-stage illnesses who want to become pregnant. Concurrent chemoradiation is the gold standard of treatment for more severe illness.

Differential Diagnosis

It's crucial to check for cervical cancer in visible cervical lesions. Yet, the majority of cervical cancers are asymptomatic and do not initially show an obvious lump. Sexually transmitted diseases, cervical fibroids, endometriosis, and cervical polyps are some more potential causes of cervical lesions or irregular bleeding. If cervical cancer is suspected, more testing and symptom analysis may be necessary for the diagnosis. A diagnostic biopsy may be required in some circumstances to provide the final diagnosis. Occasionally, a simple pap screening may reveal metastatic cancer on the uterine cervix.

Dr. Thomas H. Osborn

Chapter 3

Surgical Oncology

Cervical Cancer Surgery

Patients with cervix-confined early-stage illness are frequently given surgical resection. It can include extreme hysterectomy and somewhat benign procedures like cervical conization. Among younger individuals who want to preserve ovarian function and/or fertility, surgery is the primary treatment option for early-stage cervical malignancies.

Surgery Types

• Cervical Conization

Patients with Stage IA1 invasive cervical cancer or carcinoma in situ (CIS) illness are often candidates for cervical conization. The transformation zone and a part of the cervix can be removed using a cold knife cone (CKC), leaving at least a 3mm margin. This operation could include the use of a laser or a scalpel. It is crucial to perform a pathologic assessment of the margins and check for lymphovascular invasion (LVI). If one of these characteristics is present, further resection or a more intrusive surgical procedure may be necessary. It is pointless to perform a nodal examination if there is no LVI present on the samples since lymph node involvement is so uncommon. Patients may be seen who have negative pathologic results. Recurrence rates are normally around 10%, although they must be continuously monitored with routine cytology and colposcopy. Almost 95% of people survive for five years. Hemorrhage, infection, infertility, cervical incompetence, and stenosis are some of the complications. Complication rates vary from 2 to 12%.

• Radical Trachelectomy

Individuals who want to preserve their fertility but are not candidates for conization have undesirable clinical characteristics or more severe illnesses and might have a radical trachelectomy. The bulk of the cervix is removed during the surgery, along with the parametria, and the ureters, bladder, and rectum are all mobilized. To allow for the insertion of a cerclage to enable future pregnancy, a 5mm segment of the cervix is maintained. Because of the increased possibility of nodal involvement, a lymph node examination, including either a sentinel node biopsy or pelvic lymphadenectomy, often follows a radical trachelectomy. Adjuvant radiation with or without chemotherapy would be required if the patient had negative margins, parametria involvement, lymph node involvement, or satisfied the Sedlis criteria. Although a laparotomy or vaginal approach can be employed, there is a dearth of information about minimally invasive procedures. The overall survival rate is 97%, with a 5-year recurrence rate of about 5%. [16] Pregnancy rates after surgery are 24%, and 75% of patients give birth to living children. Issues with cervical sutures, dysmenorrhea, isthmic stenosis, and vaginal discharge are complications.

• Extra-fascial hysterectomy

The clinical grounds for extra fascial hysterectomies sometimes referred to as Type A radical hysterectomies, are limited.

Patients with Stage IA1 illness who are not interested in fertility preservation are typically offered it. It entails the complete removal of the uterus and cervix. The removal of the ovaries is not necessary with this treatment; therefore, ovarian function can be maintained. There are no parametria resection. Laparotomy or a vaginal route are both options. Evaluations of the lymph nodes are normally postponed until harmful pathologic abnormalities are found after surgery. Patients may need a full parametrectomy or external beam radiation with or without chemotherapy if it is discovered that they have unfavorable pathologic characteristics.

• Radical hysterectomy

When fertility preservation is not a top concern, a radical hysterectomy may be an option in virtually all patients with early-stage cervical cancer. The Querleu-Morrow classification has superseded the earlier Piver-Rutledge-Smith classification, which streamlined the classification procedure by basing it exclusively on the degree of lateral parametria resection. From Type A through Type D, four variations of radical hysterectomy are described. Whereas Type D reflects resections of the para cervix to the pelvic sidewall, Type A simply represents a modest parametrial resection. The two types of radical hysterectomies that are performed most frequently are Type B and Type C, which vary in that the para cervix is cut at either the level of the ureter or the internal iliac arteries, respectively. In terms of disease-free survival (91.2 vs. 97.1) and overall survival (93.8 vs. 99%), minimally invasive techniques have been demonstrated to be less effective than more well-established open procedures, with the majority of patients having Stage IB1 illness. Complications include bleeding, infection, venous thromboembolism, pulmonary embolus, small intestinal obstruction, vesicovaginal fistula, hydronephrosis, ureteral damage, stress incontinence, and lower extremities edema.

• Assessment of lymph nodes

The identification of lymph node involvement is crucial because it provides critical prognostic data and directs treatment choices. The likelihood of nodal involvement, which depends on the stage, should be taken into consideration while deciding whether to assess the lymph nodes (See Table Below). By stage, the PA nodal risk is often equal to the pelvic nodal risk. Sentinel node

Dr. Thomas H. Osborn

biopsies may also be used in certain early Stage I cervical cancer cases; however, pelvic lymphadenectomies are still the preferred procedure. Biopsies of sentinel nodes are practical and safe. With a sensitivity of 92%, a negative predictive value of 98.2%, decreased lymphatic morbidity, and no changes in recurrence-free survival, they have been studied in Stage IA1-IIA1 patients. In SENTICOL III, large-scale worldwide studies are still investigating the sentinel node biopsy method.

Dr. Thomas H. Osborn

Chapter 4

Recurring Disease

• Pelvic Exenteration

The most extreme surgical treatment for cervical cancer is pelvic exenteration. Patients with central pelvic recurrence after radiation or Stage IVA patients who cannot get radiotherapy are the only ones who qualify for indications. The removal of the uterus, fallopian tubes, ovaries, vagina, bladder, urethra, and rectum are all traditionally included in a total pelvic exenteration. A double-barrel wet colostomy, ilial conduit, or continent diversion is used for the urinary system during reconstruction, while an end colostomy or double-barrel wet colostomy is used for the GI system. Myocutaneous flaps or split-thickness skin grafts with omental J-flaps can be used to form a neovagina. Anterior and posterior exenterations, which spare the rectum or the bladder, respectively, are variations of this method. Depending on whether the urogenital diaphragm and levator muscles are removed, exenteration can also be divided into supra and infra levator categories. If a colonic anastomosis can develop, the posterior supra levator exenteration method offers the chance of preserving both urine and fecal continence. Patients who had exenteration treatment had a 40–50% five-year survival rate in recurring cases. Local recurrence rates are 84% and 75%, respectively, at 3 and 5 years. The method of execution of the exenteration has little bearing on survival. For the past 70 years, there has been a sharp decline in post-operative mortality to less than 5%, while surgical morbidity remains around 50%. Fistulas, urine leakage, peritonitis, stoma necrosis, flap necrosis, and stump dehiscence are examples of early complications. Stoma stenosis, incontinence, hydronephrosis, stone formation, and abdominal wall hernia are examples of late problems.

Pregnancy and Cervical Cancer

One of the most frequent malignancies seen during pregnancy is cervical cancer. In terms of staging and treatment, treating cervical cancer in pregnant individuals presents special difficulties. Regardless of their decision, patients should be assessed by a maternal-fetal medicine expert to facilitate discussion of risks to the fetus and probable pregnancy loss. Women must balance the risks of starting therapy right away vs. Waiting till after birth.

The gestational age must be determined. Although there is a high chance of newborn mortality and long-term damage in those who survive, the minimum fetal viability is around 24 weeks gestation. With 4% of children born at 22 weeks compared to 78% of those born at 28 weeks gestation, disability-free survival at 25 years improves significantly with later gestational ages. For comparison, the disability-free survival rate for full-term newborns is 97%.

Dr. Thomas H. Osborn

Ionizing radiation should be used sparingly in imaging investigations in this population, even if the radiation from a PET/CT scan is still much below the level needed to cause birth abnormalities and pregnancy loss.

When appropriate, it is preferable to use other imaging modalities like ultrasonography and MRI to assess the size of the local tumour and any involvement from distant metastases. Nevertheless, tiny nodal metastases are difficult to detect with MRI and ultrasound.

The use of more intrusive staging methods may be necessary. Laparoscopic pelvic lymphadenectomy may be used in a few patients with a high risk of nodal metastasis to determine the stage. While this operation may be done in any trimester and at any gestational age, it has only been investigated for safety in a small number of case studies. In some situations where sophisticated imaging is unavailable or inappropriate, these approaches may still be used. Moreover, the FIGO staging approach still permits the local staging of cervical cancer using proctosigmoidoscopy and cystoscopy (FIGO System).

Dr. Thomas H. Osborn

In a multidisciplinary setting, individualized treatment plans must be addressed with medical oncology, radiation oncology, OB-GYN, maternal-fetal medicine, and gynecologic oncology. It is initially necessary to determine the gestational age and stage of individuals who want to keep their pregnancy and get treatment. Radiotherapy is generally not recommended since the ionizing radiation dose will always result in prenatal death or serious birth abnormalities. Conization is a common therapeutic option for women with gestational ages 22 weeks and Stage IA1 illness, albeit it includes a 15% risk of substantial bleeding and spontaneous miscarriage. If the patient has an early-stage condition, gestational ages >22 weeks may be able to postpone therapy until birth. Individuals with more advanced illnesses (IB1 or greater) may have surgical resection after platinum-based neoadjuvant chemotherapy (cisplatin/paclitaxel) administration. The scant evidence points to this regimen's safety for both mother and fetus. Little series show a tumour response rate of about 75%, with local recurrences occurring in 15% of patients. These regimens include an uncertain risk of prenatal toxicity, including pediatric cancer, deformities, and respiratory distress syndrome.

Therapy should start immediately in situations of confirmed lymph node metastases, illness progression, or if the patient chooses to abort the pregnancy.

Dr. Thomas H. Osborn

The guidelines for definitive therapy are the same as those for a patient who is not pregnant if the patient discontinues the pregnancy before receiving treatment.

Part - 2

RADIOTHERAPY

Radiation is still an essential part of cervical cancer treatment. The use of radiation in practically all aspects of treatment has been proven by randomized research from the 1990s and early 2000s. Based on platinum, it can be used as a curative or adjuvant therapy, with or without chemotherapy.

Permanent radiotherapy

• Cervical Cancer in its Early Stage

early-stage cervical carcinoma IA1-IIA1, radiotherapy may the only treatment method. Compared to radical rectomy, external beam radiation with a brachytherapy offers a similar 5-year and 20-year overall survival rate d 75%, respectively) with less morbidity. Adjuvant my, however, can be possible for individuals with s >4 cm.

l cancer that has spread.

e and/or node-positive illness is often treated d chemoradiotherapy that is definitively concurrent, followed by an additional brachytherapy boost. Comparing definitive radiation with chemotherapy has significantly improved overall survival compared to radiotherapy alone, with an 8-year overall survival rate of 41% against 67%. Improvements in distant metastasis and local recurrence have also been documented.

• After-surgery radiotherapy

When particular surgical pathologic findings are present, radiation with or without chemotherapy is advised in the post-operative environment. These elements are believed to raise the chance of recurrence.

In the past, the Sedlis criteria guided the use of adjuvant radiation without chemotherapy in patients who had undergone radical hysterectomy and had at least two of the following three characteristics: >4 cm tumour size, LVSI, or >1/3 stromal invasion. These criteria were designed to identify individuals who had a 30% or greater chance of relapsing at three years. Individuals who satisfied these requirements and received pelvic radiation showed improvements in both local recurrence (21% vs. 14%) and progression-free survival (78% vs. 65%). More recently, there have been worries that the criteria's high threshold may prevent them from identifying women who may benefit from adjuvant radiation. In order to give a more linear and continuous risk assessment rather than a single threshold, a

Dr. Thomas H. Osborn

nomogram has been devised that incorporates the original Sedlis criteria as well as tumour histology.

The Peters experiment, which randomly assigned patients with positive nodes, implicated parametria, or positive surgical margins to radiation alone or with concomitant platinum-based chemotherapy, was traditionally used to suggest the inclusion of chemotherapy in radiotherapy. Chemotherapy was added, and after four years, both overall survival and progression-free survival improved by 10% and almost 20%, respectively. More recent research, including the STARS study, has aimed to increase the use of chemotherapy as an adjuvant treatment in patients who satisfy the initial Sedlis or Peters criteria.

• Delivery Methods

External beam radiotherapy, which targets the primary and pelvic lymphatics, and brachytherapy, which involves placing a sealed radiation source near the tumour, are the two main delivery techniques.

• Radiotherapy using an external beam (EBRT)

Techniques for external beam radiation include intensity-modulated radiotherapy and 3D conformal radiotherapy (IMRT). It is possible to use the intact cervical cancer sufferers' strategy. With the use of IMRT in both the adjuvant and definitive context, there has been evidence of a decrease in gastrointestinal and hematological adverse effects.

• Brachytherapy (BT)

When treating more advanced conditions, brachytherapy can be used with external beam radiation or used alone to treat early-stage conditions. The dosage delivery for this highly conformal treatment method is managed by modifying the dwell periods inside the delivery device. Further information about this method will be included in the section on brachytherapy.

• Simulation

Patients receiving external beam therapy may be positioned supine. While employing IMRT, it's very crucial to consider cervical motion. This is done by scanning the patients twice, once with a full bladder and once with an empty one. A belly board can also be used for prone placement; however, IMRT might not be repeatable if there are significant daily fraction shifts. While employing IMRT, a prone stance can provide a decrease in small bowel radiation.

Objective Delineation

On 2D x-rays, the pelvic fields—AP/PA and opposed lateral fields—were traditionally drawn to form the four-field box. The bottom of L4 served as the superior boundary of the field, and it was inferiorly drawn to the bottom of the obturator foramen, or at least 3 cm below the disease's lowest point. The front border of the lateral fields is the anterior pubic symphysis, whereas the posterior border is the sacral hollow, which includes S2.

The gross illness and elective volumes can be more precisely defined in the age of CT-based planning, PET/CT fusions, and IMRT. Gross illness detected by CT scan, PET, and physical examination would comprise a GTV. It is also possible to use an internal target volume (ITV); however, doing so would need the patient to undergo two CT simulations (empty and full bladder). The whole cervix and uterus would be covered by the CTV1 enlargement (if intact). On the main illness, PTV1 is generally 1.5 cm. The parametrial tissue, paravaginal tissues, and at least half of the upper vagina would all be included in the CTV2. Consideration should be made to covering the whole vagina if there is vaginal involvement. The recommended PTV2 enlargement is 1.0 cm. The obturator nodes, external iliac nodes,

Dr. Thomas H. Osborn

internal iliac nodes, and presacral nodes should be included in the CTV3's elective nodal volumes. If there is less vaginal involvement, consideration should be made to covering the inguinal nodes. The average PTV expansion on the elective nodes is 0.7 cm.

If there is evidence of illness in the nodal chain or the patient has a positive pelvic node and will not be getting systemic therapy, coverage of the Para aortic nodes may be necessary. The nodal strip would therefore finish at the apex of the pelvic field, L5/S1, and the superior boundary would change to the T12/L1 interspace.

Part - 3

Dosage & Dose Restrictions

The typical dosage for the entire pelvis is 45–50 Gy in 1.8–2.0 Gy fractions. If OAR limitations are not exceeded, any gross nodal illness may be increased to 60Gy.

With the implementation of intensity-modulated radiation treatment (IMRT), external beam radiation therapy has significantly improved, resulting in a decrease in acute toxicity while preserving oncologic results. The rectum, bladder, colon, femoral heads, and bone marrow are typical organs that are in danger. QUANTEC dosage limits are a great starting point. Generally, dosages of 45–50 Gy by themselves with external beam treatment will not result in appreciable rates of bladder or bowel acute toxicity. Trial methods frequently allow for rectum V4080% and bladder V4535%. Minimizing these doses during the external beam phase of treatment, if brachytherapy is intended, will enable greater doses to be administered during the boost phase of treatment. The section on brachytherapy will include dose restrictions. With the use of image-guided radiation and IMRT, bone marrow suppression resulting in Grade 3 neutropenia has been demonstrably reduced (8.6% vs 27.1%). The V1090%, V2075%, and V4037% limitations are the most typical ones for bone marrow in the pelvis. [37] [38] QUANTEC mentions V45195cc for the small bowel but more recent standards call for V4030%.

• Brachytherapy

In Stage IB2-IVA cervical cancer, brachytherapy is frequently used as a boost strategy. It permits the administration of a highly conformal dosage to the tumour while limiting exposure to healthy tissues. The most widely used approach is high dosage rate (HDR) brachytherapy (>12Gy/hr); however, it needs a radioactive source, often Iridium-192.

• Procedure

Brachytherapy is often initiated either after the external beam component of the treatment is finished or combined with EBRT during the final week of the procedure. The administration of EBRT with brachytherapy on the same day is not advised. Brachytherapy and EBRT together should not last more than eight weeks. A 1%/day decrease in local control and overall survival can be caused by prolonged treatment periods.

• Pre-implant

Dr. Thomas H. Osborn

Before conducting brachytherapy, a review of the patient's history, pathology, imaging, and physical exam should be undertaken; within a week following the surgery, a full blood and metabolic panel should be collected. Before the surgery, metabolic imbalances should be looked into and treated. Patients should wait to have the treatment done if their Absolute Neutrophil Counts (ANC) are below 500 mm. It is important to review all drugs, especially anticoagulants, and to have a PT/INR. Holding anticoagulant drugs before the operation should be carefully considered. If a patient is being treated at home, thromboprophylaxis and calf compression devices should be administered. Before the surgery, the patient should go over the bowel preparation.

• **Applicators**

There are several applicators that may be utilized in a variety of therapeutic situations. The most popular method for treating intact cervical carcinoma is the ring and tandem. The ring is inserted into the vaginal fornices while the tandem is positioned in the cervical canal. Tandem and ovoids are applied in a similar fashion but are favoured in individuals with a barrel-shaped cervix. Patients with severe parametria involvement, pelvic sidewall involvement, lower vaginal involvement, or vaginal cuff recurrence might employ interstitial applicators like the

Syed template. In situations of vaginal stenosis, difficulty inserting a ring or ovoid, or lower vaginal involvement less than 5mm thick, tandem and cylinder applicators may be employed. To provide room for interstitial needles, the Tandem and Ring or Vaginal cylinder can be modified.

• Anesthesia.

Distress for the patient and less-than-ideal applicator placement might result from the discomfort of the patient during the process. Usually, anesthetics are used to improve patient comfort and the mechanics of the treatment. General anesthesia, spinal anesthesia, epidural anesthesia, intravenous conscious sedation, and oral painkillers are some of the several forms of anesthesia that may be used.

• Placing an Intracavitary Applicator for a Cervical Intactness.

The patient is positioned in stirrups in the dorsal lithotomy posture. When the region has been sufficiently sterilized, a Foley catheter is placed, and the balloon is filled with diluted contrast to enable the detection of CT. The cervix is then seen using a speculum, and the length of the cavity is then measured using a uterine sound. This will make it easier to calculate the tandem's length and angle. In certain cases, a Smitt sleeve is utilized to preserve the cervical os's patency; however, if one is absent, serial dilations may be necessary. The tandem and ring or ovoid are then inserted when this is finished. In order to highlight the extent of the illness or the opening of the cervical os so that it is apparent on CT, fiducial markers may also be put at the time of the surgery. These applicators can be locked in place to prevent them from shifting in relation to one another.

For the purpose of lowering the excess dosage and limiting toxicity, bladder and rectum displacement is essential. One option for the packing material is gauze soaked in a radiopaque liquid. There are also available separate rectal blades or applicators with inflated balloons. The bladder is displaced by anterior packing, whereas the rectum is displaced by posterior packing. The dosage will be greatly reduced if packing is positioned in front of the ring or ovoids; hence this must be avoided at all costs.

After that, a CT simulation will be performed on the patient for 3D brachytherapy planning. When compared to 2D planning, three-dimensional CT-based planning has been demonstrated to have higher overall survival (65% vs. 74%) and reduced incidence of Grade 3–4 toxicity (23% vs. 3%). Slices should have a thickness of 1 to 5 mm. Recent advancements in planning have included the use of MRI-guided brachytherapy to provide better tissue delineation, which is best seen on T2 weighted fat-suppressed sequences (T2-FSE) imaging.] Sagittal pictures, as well as paraxial and paracoronal images, should be taken with regard to the cervix-uteri. It may also make it possible to gauge a patient's response to chemoradiation. Technically, MRI machines with low and high magnetic fields can be used. To minimize bowel motion before an MRI, patients can be given glucagon. It is advised to use a pelvic coil to improve the signal-to-noise ratio. To increase the identification of parametrial involvement, the slice thickness should ideally be 3mm, while 5mm is acceptable. This method's drawbacks include higher prices, longer operation times, and the requirement that all components be strictly MR-compatible.

Confirm that the applicator is positioned correctly. This can be done using standard radiography or more sophisticated imaging techniques like CT or MRI. In order for a tandem to be placed properly, it must bisect the ring/ovoids on AP and lateral imaging, be 1/3 to ½ the distance between the sacral promontory and the pubic symphysis, has its tip below the sacral promontory, have no packing above the ring/ovoids, and have no inferior displacement of the ring/ovoids in relation to the flange.

• Objective Delineation

The contouring of the objectives is crucial to 3D-based planning. Regarding target delineation, GEC-ESTRO has produced standardized nomenclature. The entire cervix and all gross disease are included in the high-risk clinical target volume (HR-CTV) at the start of brachytherapy treatment, the entire uterus, the upper vagina, the entire parametria, and the spaces between the bladder and rectum are included in the low-risk clinical target volume (LR-CTV), and the gross disease is also included in the intermediate-risk clinical target volume (IR-CTV) before any treatment.

Contoured normal organs at risk (OARs) should encompass the vagina, rectum, bladder, and sigmoid colon.

• Dosage Limitations and Dose.

It has been demonstrated that ensuring the target receives an appropriate dosage improves local control and survival. Depending on institutional preferences, several dosage and fractionation strategies may be used, but they must provide an 85Gy or greater total equivalent dose in two gray fractions (EQD2), assuming that 45Gy was initially administered to the pelvis. The EQD2 may be calculated using a number of different calculators. The EMBRACE trial group's EQD2 spreadsheet, often known as the "Vienna Spreadsheet," enables EQD2 calculations for the target structures and the organs at risk. The most popular dose fractionation strategies are 4 X 7 Gy, 5 X 6 Gy, and 6 X 5 Gy, with respective EQD2 values of around 90.1, 88.6, and 83.7 Gy.

The D9090% is the crucial dosimetric parameter for 3D-based planning. The aim is to cover 90% of the HR-CTV with at least 90% of the prescribed dosage. To be sure that the total dose received is 85 Gy or above, the EQD2 should be computed. In some circumstances, a modest decrease in EQD2 is appropriate. When there is a full response prior to brachytherapy or a partial response with less than 4 cm of residual illness, EQD2 > 80, Gy may be utilized, whereas more than 4 cm of residual disease is advised to use EQD2 > 85 Gy.

Even though brachytherapy treatment has continued to advance and 3D-based volumetric planning has been used, 2D dosimetric reporting methods still exist and need to be understood. The Manchester method initially included Point A, which is where the uterine artery crosses the ureter and is situated 2 cm above the tandem and 2 cm normal to the tandem. A beginning point where dosage coverage may be further adjusted in 3D to guarantee coverage of the HR-CTV, this location was generally where the prescription dose was provided in previous years. Point B, which was also a component of the original Manchester method, is situated 5 cm from the patient's midline and 2 cm up the tandem. This stands for lymphatics along the side of the pelvis, and it normally receives one-third of the prescribed dosage. It is no longer reported since it has lost popularity. For conventional tandem and ring/ovoid implants, the isodose lines should have a pear-shaped appearance. The ICRU 38 also designated a bladder and rectal point. The bladder point is situated behind the foley balloon, which has been lowered to the bladder neck. The distance between the rectal tip and the vaginal wall is 5 mm.

Doses to OARs also need to be meticulously recorded. Once more, the crucial factor is the cumulative dosage of EQD2. A brachytherapy plan is frequently assessed using the dosimetric parameter D, which measures the maximum dosage received by two cubic centimeters of tissue. The D2cc of the bladder may get up to 90 Gy EQD2, whereas the Dof rectum and sigmoid should only receive up to 75 Gy EQD2, according to the ABS standards. Recent findings, however, indicate that even with a D2cc 65Gy, late rectal morbidity may be significantly reduced.

- ## **Complications.**

Each patient receiving radiation therapy should be aware of the possibility of long-term harm. Bowel/rectal and urine problems occur most frequently. Age does not appear to have any bearing on the incidence or seriousness of problems. Within three years of therapy, there is often the highest risk of late sequelae.

Proctitis

Tenesmus and sporadic intestinal hemorrhage are side effects of radiation proctitis. Acute proctitis that might develop following radiation therapy is treated in the same way. It may take years to develop, although it normally starts to happen 3 months after therapy at the earliest. In order to reduce discomfort and halt any bleeding, treatments like mesalamine or steroid-based suppositories may be used. Randomized studies have indicated that steroid-based suppositories may not be as effective as mesalamine. The application of 4% formaldehyde can be used as another therapy to stop rectal bleeding. Argon plasma laser coagulation on the problematic vessels may be used in refractory instances.

Cystitis

Urinary frequency, hematuria, and dysuria are all symptoms of radiation cystitis. From 2-3 weeks after the commencement of radiation to 3 years afterward, it might happen suddenly.

A urinalysis is a good initial step in determining whether someone has acute cystitis in order to rule out a urinary tract infection. For dysuria alleviation, a short course of pyridium can be utilized, but the urine color change may be disconcerting for some individuals, and they should be warned ahead of time. Anticholinergic medications, such as oxybutynin or mirabegron, can be used to treat frequent urination, but older people should exercise caution while using these medications.

There is a 5–10% incidence of chronic cystitis.

Together with frequency and dysuria, these individuals are more prone to have hematuria. Mild to severe and even fatal levels of severity can exist. Patients with minor symptoms may be handled conservatively. It is important to examine and consider the patient's use of any antiplatelet or anticoagulant drugs. A cystoscopy with clot extraction and irrigation is required in more serious situations. During a cystoscopy, formalin injection

Hyperbaric oxygen treatment (HBOT) has been used in refractory instances and has been demonstrated to relieve symptoms and control bleeding in 92% of cases, while recurrences may occur.

There is also the danger of barotrauma connected with this surgery.

Second-degree cancer

Cancers brought on by radiation typically develop decades after therapy. Compared to patients who just have surgery, individuals who receive pelvic radiation have a higher overall chance of developing subsequent cancer. Under-50 treated women had a 40-year cumulative risk of 22% compared to over-50 treated women's risk of 16%. Cancers that were more common tended to affect the rectum, bladder, lung, and genitalia. Several retrospective investigations have shown an increase in leukemia incidence, which peaks approximately 5-10 years post-treatment. Reducing OAR dosages might aid in lowering the danger.

Hormonal imbalance

Ovarian failure brought on by radiation usually happens 6 to 12 months after treatment. Age-dependent minimum doses for ovarian failure range from 20.3Gy at birth to 14.3Gy at 30. It is simple to cause ovarian failure with the dosages used to treat cervical cancer. Pre-menopausal patients have some alternatives for maintaining ovarian function, including ovarian translocation or final surgery. Ovaries can be positioned 3.0 cm away from

the radiation area using laparoscopic ovarian transpositions. The preservation of fertility can also benefit from this therapy. The percentage of functional retention is about 80%.
Cryopreservation of ovarian tissue is an additional method that may be used. To avoid osteoporosis and osteopenia and to preserve libido, exogenous hormonal therapy with estrogen should be taken into consideration.

Vaginal Stenosis

After therapy, vaginal stenosis and canal shortening may appear months to years later. Stenosis can make getting gynecological checkups and having sexual activity challenging. Although regular use of a vaginal dilator is commonly advised, compliance varies greatly. It's fairly typical for people to experience sexual dysfunction, ranging from inadequate vaginal lubrication to a lack of sexual desire.

Bone fracture/ breakage

The majority of pelvic fractures are caused by dose levels of 45–63Gy in pelvic radiotherapy, which can increase the risk of pelvic fractures. Another issue for people receiving radiation to the pelvis is their bone health. A pelvic fracture occurred in around 10% of cervical cancer patients who received radiation.

Dr. Thomas H. Osborn

The sacrum is the location of fracture most frequently, and the majority of these fractures happen within two years after therapy. Scans for bone mineral density and the right treatment to preserve bone health may assist to lower this risk.

Perforation of the uterus

Uterine perforations are a brachytherapy-related problem that can lead to excessive doses being administered to healthy tissues, inadequate target coverage, bleeding, and infection. Perforation rates range from 2-18%. Controversial management options include delaying the treatment to allow for recovery or even stopping it. Delays in medical care, however, are known to have a negative impact on the result. When a blunt object causes the hole, the risk of vascular and organ harm is low; hence management of the perforation is normally expectant. Those who are stable and show no evidence of infection may be released and under watch. Antibiotics for prevention may be prescribed. Infection and signs of hemodynamic instability call for more severe treatments such as IV fluids, antibiotics, and surgical investigation.

Part - 4

Medical therapy.

Definitive

The effectiveness of platinum-based chemotherapy regimens was proven by the RTOG studies. Compared to radiation alone, there are advantages in terms of local control, overall survival, and survival without illness. Chemotherapy is thought to work as a radiosensitizer. The most often utilized drug is 40mg/week of cisplatin. As compared to non-platinum-based regimens, single-agent platinum-based regimens had the greatest progression-free survival and overall survival rates. They also had a superior toxicity profile than platinum-based regimen combos like Cis/5-FU/hydroxyurea. In situations when cisplatin would not be tolerated, carboplatin may also be utilized. Cisplatin and 5-FU are still used in several clinical settings. This treatment plan is administered alongside radiation.

Adjuvant If the patient has high-risk characteristics, chemotherapy may be added following surgical resection (Please see the radiation oncology section for more details). In some high-risk post-operative patients, the addition of chemotherapy to radiation has been shown to improve both overall survival and progression-free survival.

In clinical studies, the application of adjuvant chemotherapy following definitive chemoradiation is still being studied. Mixed outcomes have been obtained. The addition of adjuvant carboplatin/taxol to chemoradiation for locally advanced cervical cancer resulted in greater rates of grade 3-5 toxicity and no difference in overall survival or progression-free survival. An enhanced 3-year progression-free survival was seen in a study that included concurrent and adjuvant cisplatin/gemcitabine; however, the rates of grade 3–4 toxicity and hospitalizations were noticeably greater. The use of adjuvant cisplatin/paclitaxel in high-risk post-operative patients is being studied in the ongoing study RTOG 0724. (NCT00980954).

• Metastasis and Recurrence

Patients who cannot undergo reconstructive surgery or radiation in the case of recurring or metastatic disease may only get systemic treatment. Although many of these patients have already had cisplatin-based single-agent treatment, multidrug regimens are frequently employed. Patients with recurrent cervical cancer treated with cisplatin/paclitaxel have exhibited improved progression-free survival, but there was no difference in median overall survival. Other medication combinations, including cisplatin/topotecan, cisplatin/gemcitabine, and cisplatin/vinorelbine, are possible choices, but according to

GOG 204, they are not as effective as cisplatin/paclitaxel. Bevacizumab and other VEGF receptor antagonists have been added to standard chemotherapy regimens, and this has improved overall survival. For patients with a Combined Positive Score of >=1, PD-1 blockade immunotherapy has also been integrated into chemotherapy regimens and is advised. Patients with recurrent or metastatic cervical cancer have an objective response rate of 12–14% when treated with a single drug of pembrolizumab. Pembrolizumab was added to combination treatment, as shown by Keynote 826, which increased both overall survival and progression-free survival.

• Complications

Cisplatin and carboplatin are the two most widely prescribed platinum medications. Neutropenia, thrombocytopenia, anemia, febrile illness, neutropenia, nephrotoxicity, neurotoxicity, and infection are typical adverse effects. Although cisplatin is the treatment of preference, individuals who may not take cisplatin, particularly if they already have underlying renal impairment, might be treated with carboplatin. Prospective findings indicate non-inferiority in terms of efficacy despite being assumed to have reduced efficacy and a statistically significant decreased

Dr. Thomas H. Osborn

incidence of febrile neutropenia, neutropenia, and creatinine elevation.

In pre-menopausal women, bevacizumab increased the incidence of hypertension, bleeding, thromboembolic events (5% arterial and 11% venous), renal damage, and ovarian failure. Pneumonitis, colitis, hepatitis, nephritis, and endocrinopathies are among the autoimmune manifestations that pembrolizumab has been shown to precipitate.

• **Staging.**

The most widely used staging approach continues to be the International Federation of Gynecology and Obstetrics (FIGO) staging system, which had a recent upgrade in 2018. Although the TNM classification system in the AJCC 8 addition features T stages that correlate to FIGO stages, it is not frequently employed. In the past, cystoscopy, proctoscopy, hysteroscopy, urography, and plain film X-rays would all be used in conjunction with a clinical examination for FIGO staging. These very simple tests were permitted so that underdeveloped nations with limited access to healthcare could stage patients appropriately. Advanced imaging methods like MRI and PET have more recently been incorporated into the staging workup. Since MRI provides improved tissue delineation compared to CT with contrast, it is favoured for determining the T stage. The cervix is the only part of the body where FIGO stage I illness is present, and the A/B classification denotes an invasion depth of 5mm or >5mm. Stage II of the FIGO denotes illness that has spread past the uterus but not yet reached the lower vagina. The participation of the parametria has led to the A/B categorization for this stage as well. FIGO stage III refers to a disease that has spread to the lower part of the vagina (IIIA), the pelvic side wall, and/or hydronephrosis (IIIB). The nodal disease has been demonstrated to be one of the most significant prognostic markers for decreased 5-year overall survival, despite the fact that nodal disease traditionally had no impact on the FIGO staging system. The stages IIIC1 and IIIC2 were consequently created to represent the involvement of the para-aortic nodes or pelvic nodes, respectively. FIGO Stage IVA illness denotes a locally aggressive condition that has affected nearby organs like the bladder or rectum or has spread beyond the actual pelvis. FIGO stage IVB illness shows non-regional nodal disease or metastasis to other solid organs.

• Prognosis

The HPV vaccine is thought to be 90% effective. An independent risk factor for cervical cancer diagnoses that are made too late is inconsistent screening. Cervical cancer has a survival rate of up to 92 percent after five years. The likelihood of recurrence increases, and survival falls with a greater presentation stage. Black American women often have the lowest survival rates and highest death rates. It's possible that less than 50% of people will survive. The administration of

Dr. Thomas H. Osborn

evidence-based therapy, lymph node spreading, age, and the size and invasion of the tumour at the time of diagnosis are all potential contributing factors to variations in outcomes.

Advanced cancer complications and their related therapies are comparable to those of other malignancies. Renal failure, hydronephrosis, discomfort, lymphedema, bleeding issues, and fistulas are possible complications. Please see the sections on each treatment option for further information on the unique problems of the various treatments.

• **Patient Education and Dissuasion**

Both conventional and cutting-edge patient education strategies can raise awareness of cervical cancer and the need for early detection and prevention. According to the research, clinicians might not be discussing or suggesting HPV vaccination with patients. Parents and women both worry about vaccinations. More training for doctors in high-risk communities may improve screening, prevention, and awareness among the women who are most at risk for death. Nonetheless, a patient can favor the provider's explanation of the healthcare system. Through community outreach, it is necessary to increase patient education and awareness of cervical cancer prevention and screening outside of the clinical setting. This additional education should include culturally appropriate information,

Dr. Thomas H. Osborn

appropriate language to reach low health literacy populations, and targeted efforts for women who are not yet sexually active.

• Among Other Things: Pearls

Vaccination is a primary method of cervical cancer prevention. A quadrivalent vaccination exists that guards against genital warts in addition to cervical cancer. For females, the recommended age range for immunization is 9 to 45 years old. Both men and women between the ages of 9 and 45 are encouraged to use it. Health promotion focusing on vaccination can have a large influence on cervical cancer mortality in women in poor resource regions and those who are in high-risk ethnic groups. In the US, a vaccination that just protects against HPV 16 and 18 is no longer available. Its use could nonetheless continue in other nations outside the United States.

• Improving Healthcare Team Results

The prevention, screening, treatment, and management of cervical cancer can all be improved with the assistance of an interprofessional team. Public education can raise awareness of the need to recognize precancerous lesions and the necessity of cervical cancer prevention and screening. Primary care clinicians who do colposcopies, LEEP procedures, and cervical cancer screenings must regularly communicate with

Dr. Thomas H. Osborn

gynecologists regarding results, worrisome lesions, management, and therapy. Increased awareness, screening, management and treatment, and follow-up can all benefit from organized procedures and recommendations throughout the system. Diverse personnel and providers with language proficiency, cultural sensitivity, and lab and nursing expertise will also be needed to contribute to the development of a system that is culturally responsive and aims to increase patient-centered education.

By coordinating care and communication, the interprofessional team may improve the way that patients are treated. Diagnoses and treatment strategies are provided by general practitioners, gynecologists, radiation oncologists, and nurse practitioners. Oncology nurses and nurses who specialize in specialty care should collaborate with the team to coordinate treatment and be involved in patient education. The remainder of the team should receive their input. Pharmacists should assess recommended drugs and immunizations, be aware of drug-drug interactions, educate patients, and keep track of compliance. Hence, the team can enhance the prognosis for cervical cancer patients. [level 5]